The Secret Mindset for Diet

James Wallace

DEDICATION

This book is dedicated to all those readers who have followed the advice of diet and fitness experts, tried to succeed, and then failed for no fault of their own.

It's not your fault that these "influencers" were more concerned with your cash than with truly assisting you! They mishandled you, not you. To alter that, I'm here.

CONTENTS

ACKNOWLEDGMENTS

I want to express my gratitude to all of the wonderful people who have helped me get to this point. With regard to writing, editing, and releasing this book, I received some excellent guidance and assistance. This wouldn't have been possible without your assistance, so thank you!

Additionally, I'd like to thank all of the motivational colleagues I've had throughout the years. I want to thank you as well since your journeys have improved my understanding and fueled my desire to assist as many people as I can.

Finally, I'd like to express my gratitude to my loved ones. You all know who you are. I wouldn't be able to put my ideas forward and pursue my dreams without your unwavering love and support.

Chapter One
How to Start

Welcome to The Secret Mindset for a Diet, my first book ever! First off, I want to thank you for purchasing it (unless you already own an illegal copy in which case I appreciate the follow, but don't be so strict!). I'm eager to support you in changing for the better without sacrificing your way of life.

You'll note that the book isn't very long, and the reason is really straightforward: I don't have a very long attention span, so I don't see the purpose in filling up lots of pages with information that you don't really need. I like to get right to the point.

I'm going to show you how to get your motivation going so you can accomplish your goals in this book.

There is a wealth of information available on how to exercise and what foods to eat, but no one seems to explain how to become and maintain motivation to work toward your goals. Therefore, in the pages that follow, we'll examine what motivation is, what factors influence it, and how to create a strategy to maximize it for the greatest likelihood of success. We'll also examine why you respond in particular ways and what you can do to prevent it from deflecting your attention.

So let me give you a little background information on myself (spoiler alert: I didn't almost die and you won't hear a sad narrative; this book isn't that kind, and I'm not that kind of coach!) I was a contentedly overweight youngster who most likely would have remained such if it weren't for peer pressure, bullying, and other forms of harassment. At primary school, I was "large boned," as my mother would describe, but not overly overweight, so peers didn't really say anything.

Things didn't really pick up until I entered secondary school, where there was a canteen selling pizza, doughnuts, cakes, and other items, as well as an ice cream van on the playground.

Nothing made me happier than visiting my Nan on a Sunday, sipping coffee, and eating the finest biscuits! She was the best because she would keep the nice stuff a secret until I came to visit. I gained additional weight as a result of these improvements in eating, and before I realized it, I was fairly overweight.

I fell in love with rugby because I was wanted because I was fat when I discovered it in secondary school. Brilliant! I began out as a prop (the fat person in the front row of the scrum). While that was fantastic, teases had begun to surface.

My Name is James. We were fairly good friends, so even though he was small and slender and I was a big, fat boy, we frequently hung out together. Because they were too slow to explain everything, our pals decided to call me "fat James" or, and here is the irony, FJ for short, to avoid confusion. You're free to chuckle at the moniker. There were numerous comments to my weight made every day, which initially didn't bother me much but eventually became into sound effects and included people I didn't like, at which point I became upset by it. This occurred over a period of several years, during which time we grew older and our buddies began to date other people.

This is where it all began for me when I realized I had to take action. When I was at 14, I realized I needed to get my food under control and start moving my big ass! We'll examine this mindset throughout the book since it was actually quite potent. Although I had little interest in health and fitness, I was relatively clever and could figure out where my eating habits were flawed, and it was clear that I wasn't getting enough exercise. It all started there! Another spoiler alert: I didn't go on to win Mr. Olympia, and you won't find a ton of photographs of me almost completely undressed on Instagram (at least, I hope not; if there are, they'll only be rugby-related).

I'm a fairly typical guy who manages a business, maintains a healthy lifestyle, and continues to play, coach, and officiate rugby.

Having said that, the majority of my heavy lifts—bench press, squat, deadlift, etc.—are above 100 kg, and I can do a 10-kilometer run in under an hour. This is the standard by which I like to gauge my level of fitness and health. I want to be able to lift a good amount of weight, be physically capable of covering a reasonable amount of ground in a reasonable amount of time when running, and have a waist measurement that is reasonably close to my chest and shoulder measurements! This is the mindset and attitude I want to see you develop.

I won't lie to you; the fitness industry irritates me (to put it nicely). It is rife with garbage. Even with only personal trainers and facility operators, people are being deceived everywhere. You guys are even worse off if you're looking for advice and support. Don't get me wrong, there are some wonderful trainers out there who can help you achieve amazing results, but they are frequently overshadowed by show ponies who appear fantastic on the outside but won't reveal how they achieved that appearance because it would damage their credibility! Both men and women in the field should be aware of this!

You shouldn't be surprised that you're disoriented because there are so many fads, fast solutions, "experts," and "opportunities" being aggressively promoted that appear "too good to miss." Without regulation, the craziness and cowboy behavior in the fitness sector will spread and increase. Yes, they are making money. In certain cases, fairly significant sums of money, but they are given to you at your expense, ruining the standing of the industry for the rest of us! That's what I'm here for; I'll tell it like it is, and together, we'll develop a strategy for the average person. I'm probably not the coach for you if you really want abs and a cover model physique, but I have instructors who can provide you with those things. We'll talk more about this later.

The majority of this novel was written during a peculiar time in life when the majority of the world is under lockdown and hiding from Covid-19 (no pun intended). This poses several difficulties for us generally, but particularly for our food and exercise regimens. When things return to normal, there will be two outcomes for each person: person A will have been as active as possible and watched what they ate and drank, and may even have emerged in better shape. Then there is person B, who will eat or drink to pass the time when they are bored and will likely buy items that will make them feel better but also add to their body fat.

I'm going to presume that you are/have been person B since you purchased this book, but that's okay because you fall into the category of the people I'm here to assist! So let's get started based on that.

Chapter Two
Current State

There are a lot of choices and resources available in today's fitness and nutrition environment. It can be challenging to use social media and the internet without coming across the newest celebrity fitness expert or trendiest new diet. The importance of body shape and numerous methods for losing weight and becoming in shape has gained worldwide attention. That's not inherently a negative thing, but as I hinted at in the chapter before, it has led to widespread disinformation and uneducated beliefs.

Trainers and coaches must work harder to stand out as the market gets more saturated. Unfortunately, this has led to fit professionals promoting severe dieting techniques in order to produce speedy results for before-and-after images. While participants do lose weight and fat in the short term, these fast cures don't educate participants or help them mend their relationships with food, which frequently leads to a rebound when participants start eating the same way they did before.

Diets frequently ignore issues like education and mending people's relationships with food, and as I grow cynical in my outlook on life, I start to wonder whether this is just to support and sustain profit margins.

Let's examine the structure of well-known weight-loss clubs; I won't even disclose their names because I know you can name them right away. They have done a fantastic job of developing brands and gaining a huge global audience. They have also assisted a great deal of people in drastically altering their lives by helping them drop a lot of weight or fat. What occurs though if you stop going to the club and sticking to the programme? The weight or fat often returns. Although I acknowledge that not everyone experiences that, and that the most are likely still in a better position than they were initially, my argument is still that why does it happen?

Because they instruct people in following a system, rather than helping them learn about nutrition, regulate eating, emotional reactions, and change habits. Additionally, they stigmatise some meals and associate bad eating habits. Due to the worsening of the relationship with food and the increased sense of limitation, there is a higher likelihood that non-conformance will occur.

When you have anything "naughty," what happens? You feel guilty and disappointed in yourself. What follows? Oh well, I screwed up today; I might as well get what I want and start fresh tomorrow or Monday! How frequently have you stated or acted in this way?

For these reasons we must be smarter with restriction, and that's what this book is for. Restriction sounds like a horrible word, but in reality, that's what all diets are. They are dressed up and marketed in many different ways, let's look at some of the ways they do this...

Low-carb diets

Celebrities and fitness experts have demonised carbohydrates, portraying them as the enemy of weight loss. The main cause of this is that the majority of us normally eat diets high in carbohydrates. Whether it's breakfast cereal, a sandwich from the grocery store, or a burger from the takeout menu, many of the quick options we choose are carb-based. They are frequently excellent, filling, and simple. As a result, they contribute significantly to our daily calorie intake. So, if we limit our intake of carbohydrates, we inevitably consume less calories overall, which results in weight loss and fat loss. The issue with this is that we also consume significantly less energy because our body prefers to utilise carbohydrates.

Intermittent fasting

The body simply cycles through phases of fasting and feeding using this strategy. So, rather than limiting certain food groups, you now only control when you eat them. There are different time periods, yet they all ultimately lead to the same result. Again, intermittent fasting offers a technique to lower daily calorie intake because it typically results in skipping a meal, frequently breakfast. As long as they don't overeat to make up for the missed meal, this can be a useful strategy for people who don't want to strictly manage their calorie intake. For people with hectic and unpredictable days, however, confining to specific time periods throughout the day may not be the best option. For instance, those who travel

Meal replacements

This is the process of substituting bars, shakes, smoothies, etc. for meals. It is just nonsense! I apologise for being so direct, but I have very strong feelings about it. You will probably lose weight, and possibly rather quickly. What does it, however, teach you about food? Exactly nothing! How does it enable you to develop healthier attitudes around food and portion sizes? There isn't! You should avoid utilising meal replacements unless you're in a dangerous situation where you need to lose weight quickly for a medical operation!

Protein drinks should not be confused with meal substitutes. I've seen folks who struggle to eat in the morning to use protein as a means to ingest calories until they feel ready to eat, and some people use protein smoothies to boost their protein intake. That, in my opinion, is different.

What are the goals of a meal replacement plan? You guessed it—to limit calorie intake. So why in the world would you choose a meal replacement if you can do that while still enjoying your food?

Paleo diet

The term "caveman diet" is also sometimes used to describe this. It adheres to the idea that food should only be obtained from hunting, fishing, or growing. It is a naturally low-carb, high-protein diet that excludes processed food. Once you get into it, eating healthy, nutritious foods actually makes you feel wonderful, which may be quite beneficial for weight/fat loss. However, unless you are dedicated to food preparation, it can be difficult. If you are eating out or getting food on the run, it is exceedingly challenging to adhere to the rules. So, if this is your preferred diet, you must take this into account.

This strategy is also a little different because it isn't strictly calorie-controlled, but you'll still probably cut calories when you consume fewer carbohydrates, fats, and sugars.

It is a good alternative (in my opinion) if you can eat this way, but it can be time-consuming and expensive.

Therefore, all diets have the same goal of establishing a calorie deficit, regardless of whether they limit feeding times, track calories, eliminate certain food groups, etc. In an effort to persuade you that the technique they are selling is better than all others, these systems have their fan bases, which also include trainers and coaches who promote them. However, if you reverse engineer every diet, they all still have the same goal.

In actuality, it doesn't really matter what time you consume specific food types, nor does it matter if you eat everything inside a set window of time. What counts is the difference between your daily calorie intake and expenditure. You will gain weight if you consume more than you use, and you will lose weight if you utilise more than you consume. Therefore, why add unnecessary complexity by creating a long list of rules and regulations?

Food plays a significant role in daily life and greatly affects our wellbeing. Food plays a significant role in who we are and what we do, from social relationships to self-esteem and mood. Therefore, having a positive relationship with food is essential for both our physical and emotional well-being. Because of this, we must exercise caution when utilising limitation in order to both safeguard ourselves and maximise our chances of success.

It's time to throw out the systems, stop demonising meals, live guilt-free, and start moving forward effortlessly. Restraint need not equate to agony! We're going to improve our bodies while continuing to eat the things we enjoy and lead fulfilling lives!

Chapter Three

Setting a Goal: What do you actually hope to accomplish?

We will focus on what you REALLY want to accomplish in this section. I can hear you say, "I want abs." I want to appear like Zac Efron, but 1) I lack his good features and hairline, and 2) I'm not willing to make the same kind of commitment to my social life that he is. That is the situation's reality, and you must take that into account when setting a SMART objective for yourself. The success or failure of your goal will depend on a variety of elements that you must take into account while creating one.

1) Where do you want to start? You really need to be honest with yourself because this is nearly exclusively centred on your composition (body fat percentage, muscle mass, etc.). Is it reasonable to set your initial objective to acquire a six pack if you are 30 stone and 50% body fat? Without a doubt! In contrast, setting a goal to put on 5 stone of lean muscle in a year when you weigh 10 stone and have 10% body fat is similarly unattainable! The best method to destroy your motivation based on the likelihood of failure is to set impossible goals! It's acceptable to

have a large aim in mind as your ultimate objective, but you must divide it into smaller targets to accomplish along the road.

What are the focuses of your lifestyle? This is definitely very crucial! You need to think about how important such things are to you if you regularly get takeout, go out to dinner three to four times each month, or go out for drinks every weekend. If you want to keep doing those activities, that is totally acceptable, but remember to account for it when you establish your goal! I enjoy going out to eat at least once a week (during normal, non-covid times) and enjoying a drink after rugby, so I won't get into Zac Efron shape. However, I'm okay with that because I'd rather be social and in reasonable form than antisocial and look amazing. I've chosen to just go out drinking once or twice a month as of right now (when I first started in "normal times") because I've gone out too often over the past few months, it's costing me a fortune, I'm a slob with a hangover, and my body fat percentage is suffering. Having said that, I'm not ready to stop going out to eat because I like it and still want a social life! You must be honest with yourself and take responsibility for your decisions. If you have realistically and correctly planned, your outcomes shouldn't come as a surprise to you.

How frequently can you commit to working out? I'll use the phrase again, but what does "realistic" mean to you? Which type of exercise do you enjoy doing, and how frequently do you want to perform it? I'm pleased to lift weights 3–4 times each week because I find it enjoyable. I can definitely commit to walking once or twice a week because I enjoy it. I run 5 km on average while I'm in season because I play or officiate rugby at least once a week. In the off-season, I might make up for it by playing racketball or going for a run. So you would exercise about five times per week. I'm not ready to work out twice a day at this time. That is an accurate reflection. However, you also need to consider whether you can fit it in around your obligations to your family, friends, and job. There is always time for exercise, as I'm meant to remind you as a certified personal trainer, but as a mindset and motivation coach, I'm reminding you that if you're not up for it, you won't do it, so it needs to be relevant to you and your life. You can base your objective on how frequently you can commit to exercising once you've thought about these factors. It will eventually influence how quickly and how far you get to your goal.

What kind of exercise do you enjoy? This is enormous! It's very straightforward: If you don't enjoy it, you won't stick with it. It might be effective in the short run for fast wins, but since it's not a part of your long-term strategy, it's unlikely to help you reach your ultimate objective. Focus on a strategy centred around your preference for lifting weights, aerobic, or group exercise classes if you prefer them. Yes, there are some types of exercise that are more efficient or could produce effects more quickly, but in the end, this needs to be something you enjoy doing so that when the time comes to exercise, you actually do it.

What's your knowledge like?

Do you understand gym plans and exercises?

Could you download a workout plan and go and do it without help?

If the answer is yes, you know what the exercises are and can safely perform them, then go to work! It's okay if you're a newbie and you don't know anything; there's no need to feel embarrassed; just ask an expert or trained trainer for assistance. Once you have the information and a strategy, the next issue is

Can you do it by yourself?

Will you turn up 3-4 times a week?

If you've had a tough day will you still go?

This isn't a sales pitch; PTs are pricy (if a trainer is inexpensive, there's probably a good reason why; my schooling, which included an exercise science degree and a PT certification, cost somewhere over £40,000). If you can make it there on your own and are dedicated to carrying out the exercises on your plan, great! Keep going and take pleasure in the outcomes of your labour of love. You must hire a trainer or find a dedicated training partner if you are a "tomorrow" type who can easily talk yourself out of things.

Consistency is the key to getting results, with a 12-week commitment being the very minimum. However, let's face it, for most of us and our starting points (including mine), we're probably looking at a year to make the changes that we really desire. Sorry if reading that made you cry, but this book is straight-forward!

We have to account for vacations and events where we yell "f#*k it" and destroy the BBQ and bar since it takes time to break habits and change patterns! This isn't a 12-week low-carb makeover; instead, I'm assisting you in learning how to reprogramme your life. But you must understand that it will still entail eating and drinking in a different way than you are accustomed to since, let's face it, the fact that you bought this book indicates that you realise something has to change!

Having said that, there will still be occasions when you throw it all out the window and revert to typing, even though you are not on a diet. It happens. Things occur that make us unbalanced! You are in charge, and that is important! You indulge in it for the duration of the event or even for a couple of days before saying, "Okay, that was fun, but I want to get back to eating and exercising well now," and you'll do that because feeling fitter and healthier is far preferable to feeling slobby and depressed! This mindset is so effective because it prevents you from acting as though someone has just passed away and gives you control over the fact that you briefly let your guard down.

You are in charge of your outcomes now that you have chosen to stick to your original strategy. When all of this is taken into account, we're looking at a year, or longer depending on where you start. Rome wasn't created in a day, therefore it's okay! Although there are elements of science and psychology in this book, the entire thing is based on personal experience. We're in this together because the inner fat boy still battles mightily to get out every day. As a result, I understand your struggles and the advice I'm giving you is advice I also follow.

Anyway, I rambled a lot there although I hope it was useful! Back to training. There are so many different types of training

✓ Strength

✓ CrossFit

✓ Bodybuilding

✓ Powerlifting,

✓ Strongman

✓ Hiit

✓ Endurance

✓ Exercise to music and so on.

Sport is also a significant factor in health and wellness; those are just gym-based activities. My argument is that if you tell me you don't enjoy exercising, you're lying! The same way those who claim to detest fruit do! I take it you've tried every sport and form of exercise there is, and you don't enjoy any of them? If that IS the case, you are doomed to be overweight and unwell, and it is your own!

Even if you're terrible at it, there will be a game or activity that you like. Rugby is something I'm just mediocre at, but I adore it and will "ran" around a pitch for 80 minutes. Regardless of how skilled you are, it really only matters if you participate. It truly doesn't matter if you're horribly unfit or extremely overweight! Who cares if you can only bench press with 2 kg of dumbbells or can only sprint for 20 seconds before walking again? What matters is that you do it and that you continue to do it week after week until it becomes easier and you push yourself to go further or lift more weight. You are vying with yourself in this.

I can demonstrate this to you since while I was working out by myself in a chain gym and trying to complete an extra rep of the bench press because it was going well, no one even noticed, including other users and trainers passing by! Prior to being able to sit up and lift it off, I had to roll it down my body. So, no, not as many people are watching you as you might imagine.

So, with all that in mind let's look at creating you a goal to work towards. We're going to use SMART goals. Specific, Measurable, Achievable, Relevant, and Time bound.

Specific - Without further ado, what is the primary objective? Drop half a stone? Reduce your personal best time for the 5 km by 30 seconds? 105 kg bench press maximum of 1 rep? (By the way, I adore the bench press; it's my favourite exercise, and I'm not sorry for using it in all of my examples.)

Measurable - how are you going to track it? Fitness app? Workout diary? Pictures?

Achievable - Is it realistic? Have you set a goal to lose 3st in a month?

Relevant - Does it support your objective? Does it make sense in light of what your ultimate objective is? For instance, suppose you want to gain lean muscle mass but you've committed to an ironman triathlon. That's not realistic because doing cardio will burn a lot of calories, and unless you can eat like a machine and ingest a lot of calories each day, you will lose weight and muscle mass.

Time bound - Establish timelines for when you want to complete tasks. This will assist in keeping you accountable and focused. But make sure it's attainable and practical. You won't be able to reduce your waist size by 10 inches in a month. However, if losing 10 inches is your ultimate objective, you can set a monthly goal of at least one inch. It's a good idea to have a big objective and many smaller, attainable ones along the road. Achieving success is a fantastic method to increase motivation, which creates momentum. If your goals are being met and you're feeling well, you'll workout harder, eat better, feel better, and the outcomes will continue to improve!

When you break down SMART goals, it just makes sense to set them out this manner even though they have a very corporate feel to them. First off, it's a terrific technique to determine whether they are dreams or reality! Accomplish you believe "yes, I can do that" when you read it aloud to yourself? Your exam is that. If the response is a sincere "yes," you're on the right track and have moved forward in a very logical way!

The second stage is to get your brain in the correct place after you have a goal that is achievable and well-thought-out. It all depends on your mindset! To achieve growth, you must create habits that are consistent with your outlook and objectives; doing so will mean the difference between success and failure.

Chapter Four
Understanding Motivation

It's easy, right? the explanation for WHY a person does something or acts in a certain way. or the desire to do something, particularly something that requires effort and hard work.

The solution to successfully altering body shape can be summed up by those two definitions or claims. Before you can decide how much you WANT to make the change, you must first understand WHY you want to do it in the first place. Then why do we battle so much if it's that simple? To figure out how to unlock motivation and harness it to be successful, we need to understand it a little more.

Among the many variables that influence motivation, the physical and psychological environments can both have a significant impact. For instance, when you walk through a shopping centre, there are food kiosks wherever you turn, and everything smells and looks fantastic. If you dislike shopping, this situation will be made worse because it will immediately catch your attention. Even if you aren't hungry now, once you've seen everything there is, you will be. If you're with someone who doesn't share your objectives, it's quite improbable that you'll leave the centre without stopping at one of the food establishments.

Which takes us to your support system and psychological surroundings. Your likelihood of success can be significantly impacted by surrounding yourself with people who have understanding and positive attitudes. In contrast to that friend who tries to convince you to "relax" and tells you "one little meal won't hurt you," if you are with someone who understands what you want to achieve and why you want to achieve it, they are much more likely to help you make positive choices, perhaps through encouragement or even by joining in with you.

Now, I'm not saying you to weed out your friends and family if you want to succeed, but we'll talk about this again when we build a strategy to deal with these obstacles! Just remember that contextual circumstances will test your resolve and motivation, and that you must comprehend why and how to prepare to avoid being derailed.

As you might expect, there are many theories about what motivates people. The three approaches to motivation are trait-centered, situation-centered, and interactional.

According to the trait-centered view, motivation levels are influenced by a person's personality and other unique traits. According to the view, an individual's motivation originates from within rather than from outside sources. Therefore, psychologists concur that a person's motivations are greatly influenced by their personality, needs, and aspirations (Weinberg and Gould, 2007). According to me, this does not establish someone's motivation on its own. Rather, it is critical that you reflect on yourself and be truthful about your own nature. What "needs" must you have in order to succeed? Do you need a lot of "small wins" to stay motivated, or do bigger goals inspire you? This process will lead to lots of self-learning where you get closer to working out and understanding who you are and what you need to be successful. Wow we're getting deep...

According to the situation-centered view, a person's motivation is affected by the circumstances surrounding them. This may depend on an activity, location, or person and can have a positive or negative impact on your level of motivation. As opposed to attending an outdoor bootcamp in the bitter cold with a would-be Army Physical Training Instructor, you might feel more inspired to work out at the gym with your friends in a class taught by a superb instructor. In order to succeed, you'll need to learn more about yourself again and identify the situation in which you're most likely to do well. If you sign up for something that isn't really you, of course you'll find reasons not to do it. It's only normal for you to put your time and energy into the things you enjoy or are greatest at. In order to advance, you must create a situation that meets your criteria.

According to the Interactional View, performance and behaviour are strongly predicted by both personality and situation. It implies that the best performance will be determined by the personality of the person and the environment in which they work. In terms of fitness, one size doesn't really fit all. You won't necessarily get the same results as a person who adores Zumba and has lost 2 sizes since beginning. You need to think about your personality type, what you enjoy doing, where you prefer doing it, how long you have left, whether you'll be doing it with others, and if so, who. I intentionally kept that vague because the same concepts apply to both diet and exercise. Once you've resolved these issues, you may begin developing your strategy.

I keep coming back to the idea of figuring out who you are and what your needs are because it is based on two psychological principles: the desire for success and the desire for failure (Need achievement theory, McClelland, 1961; Atkinson, 1974). An individual will be motivated to either participate in (approach) or retreat from (avoid) a situation, depending on whether feeling is stronger, according to this idea, which is referred to as an approach-avoidance model. A person will be motivated to participate in a situation if they believe they have a better probability of succeeding than they have of failing. If a person's fear of failure, however, outweighs their odds of success, they will probably try to avoid or withdraw from the circumstance. Be achievement motivation is a personality attribute or a relatively constant way of acting, this technique is referred to as trait-centered. Although it's unlikely to be the only factor influencing motivation, the circumstances can alter both the likelihood of success and the motivation for it. A circumstance with a high likelihood of success and a strong payoff may encourage those who lack intrinsic motivation.

Look at that in context, shall we? Although I wouldn't describe myself as especially confident, I grew up playing rugby and am quite confident. The increase in testosterone levels has occurred frequently, and it serves as an excellent illustration of motivation. We'll use arm wrestling as an example; while I'm delighted that I'm reasonably strong, I detest appearing foolish in front of others. As a result, in this scenario, my prospects of success and my fear of failure are actually at odds with one another. Therefore, when deciding which combat to accept, I consider how sure I am in my ability to defeat the opponent. I'm more likely to accept the challenge if I believe I have a decent chance of winning and will seem good in front of my friends. However, if I don't think I can win, I'll probably take all available precautions to stay away from the conflict. We choose how we exercise in exactly the same way, whether it's which class we attend, whether we try to lift weights, whether we register for a running event, etc.

On the other hand, the idea also explains why "high achievers" seek more tough activities since they place a larger value on success if they find it more difficult. Naturally, this results from a strong sense of self-assurance, which is why they see more success as likely and like the extra challenge. That being said, even if you don't think of yourself as a "high achiever," there will still be circumstances in which you feel comfortable choosing the more difficult course of action due to your abilities and expertise!

I know theories are boring, but they will enable us to understand why we make decisions and how we come to them. Please bear with me.

To further understand ourselves and what can affect our motivation we have to look at Weiner's Attribution Theory (Weiner, 1985).

Given that most individuals want to know why things occur as a result of the outcome, it focuses on how people explain their success or failure. In general, attributes are categorised as internal or external, stable or unstable (permanent or continually changing) (within or outside of our control). Therefore, when these elements are considered together, success or failure can be attributed to skill or effort, task complexity or luck. The conclusions we get from them have a significant impact on our motivation because they have an impact on our self-confidence and expectations for future success. As a result, attributes improve our self-confidence in a particular setting by either making us feel better about ourselves or shielding us from feeling awful. As our degrees of self-confidence frequently influence whether we perform or avoid in a circumstance, this will have an impact on motivation moving ahead.

Using a real-world illustration I follow a few members of a well-known weight loss brand on social media, and every week they publish whether they've lost weight, kept the same weight, or gained weight. See where I'm going with this? Most often, the post is accompanied with an explanation. The post that kills people is one that says, "totally gutted, I've eaten really well this week and exercised, and I haven't lost anything," or anything like. The fact that weight fluctuates so much means that even when the internal part of effort is perfect, the outcome is primarily external because there is a little amount of chance involved in whether the scale reading will be different when it comes time to weigh in. You might even return the following morning lighter! In this instance, you must realise that timing, not effort level, is the true reason of your perceived failure. Keep up your consistency, and the results will come.

On the other hand, if you haven't put in the effort (internal), you can't just point to luck (external) and claim that's why; if you want to succeed, you have to be honest and consider all the variables. It's crucial that you properly evaluate your performance in order to prevent assigning blame or having your motivation suffer in the future. You should now be able to comprehend the remark "there's no use in me trying, I never lose weight anyway" and its origins after learning about these variables.

Additionally, keep in mind that on a transformation programme, remaining the same counts as progress! For the reasons mentioned above, there will be weeks when the scales remain unchanged, but consider the big picture! As long as your percentage of body fat hasn't increased, you are still further along than when you began.

Let's summarise this so we can create our strategy and determine what each of us needs in order to stay motivated. If you're listening to an audiobook, grab some paper because I'll leave space for you to take notes. Following a strategy for exercise, we'll create one for food.

Exercise

What type of exercise do you enjoy most? Cardio, Resistance, Martial Arts etc.

Environment

Where do you prefer to exercise? Home, Green Space, Gym etc.

Who do you prefer to exercise with? By yourself, in a group, with friends, with a PT.

Do you want/need competition from others or are you happy chasing your own targets?

Do you require a PT appointment, a class or boot camp appointment, or a gym companion appointment?

Can you commit to working out alone?

Frequency/Duration

How many times per week can you realistically commit to exercise?

How much time can you dedicate to exercising? Do you want to keep the weekly session lengths the same or change them up? Include it in your strategy.

Tracking

Do you want to track your exercise (time/weights/reps etc) or do you just want to enjoy a workout?

Food

What type of food do you enjoy most?

Which foods do you need to cut back on? (Notice that I didn't say cut out; we want a normal existence, just one without excess.)

Environment

Can you rely on yourself to keep these foods in your home, or do the cabinets require careful stocking?

Do you need to take food with you, or can you trust yourself not to buy excessively?

Do you need to bulk prepare your meals or can you trust yourself to cook when you get home?

Do you want/need accountability from others or are you happy chasing your own targets?

Can you prepare your own eating plan, or do you need help from a professional?

Now that we have some answers, let's hope that you have searched deeply within yourself and that your replies are totally sincere. I make an effort to avoid being snarky, but I can't help it since it keeps me entertained and since I become easily distracted, it's essential when writing a book.

Although I partially mock this, it is crucial that you have been honest with yourself. Take advantage of the chance to be really honest about your needs because this is your book and only you will see it unless you want others to. This is your time to indulge in all your selfish desires! It's all about you in this book! With this knowledge, we can develop a strong mindset that can help you achieve your goals.

Chapter Five
Make Mindset for Success

It may sound apparent, but mindset is crucial for success. Put simply, if your head isn't in it, you won't succeed! You probably already know how simple it is to lose concentration, and before you know it, you're back where you started, wondering what the heck just happened. The risky part is that every time you stray from your plan, you serve to further solidify the notion that you won't succeed in your objectives, and as a result, low self-esteem and self-doubt develop inside of you. Before you start thinking, "What's the purpose in trying?," we must take action!

We need to establish some fundamental routines that will get you out of this rut and keep you on track. You will need to repeatedly practise these skills until they sink in and your thinking naturally supports them. However, there is no reason why you won't be able to accomplish your goals if they are there and you are living by them.

In what way then do we "establish a habit"? Let's first define what a habit is. It can be characterised as an action that is automatically triggered in response to contextual factors connected to its performance (Neal, et al 2012). For instance, getting out of bed and immediately putting on clothing (contextual cue). According to a fairly broad body of research, doing the same action repeatedly in the same situation over time makes the action more likely to be engaged in response to a cue. Or, to put it another way, you learn to carry out an activity when you are in the appropriate situation after repeatedly performing a task over time.

Dependence on conscious attention or motivational processes is diminished once action initiation is "transferred" to environmental signals (Lally, Wardle and Gardner, 2011). Simply said, we stop having to think about completing the action once repetition has taught us to react to the contextual cue. When we are young, we are taught to wash our hands after using the restroom. After some time, and after receiving continuous assistance, we learn to do it without being reminded. We just wash our hands without stopping to consider it.

The most basic piece of habit-formation guidance is to continuously repeat an action in the same situation. The "initiation phase," where the new behaviour and the environment in which it will be practised are chosen, is where the habit formation effort starts. The succeeding "learning phase," in which the behaviour is repeated in the selected context to strengthen the association between the situation and the behaviour, is when automaticity emerges (here a simple tick sheet for self-monitoring performance may help). The'stability phase', where the habit has developed and reached a plateau in strength and persistence throughout time with little effort or thought, is where habit formation culminates (Gardner, Lally and Wardle 2012).

Put that into action, shall we? As I stated at the opening of the book, I am writing during the COVID-19 pandemic lockdown period. Since I can only leave the house for necessary shopping and one exercise session each day, I choose to take advantage of the situation to address my hydration. I've had a bad habit of not drinking enough water in the past, and one of my justifications is that I have to urinate A LOT when I first start hydrating, and that isn't always doable when I'm on the road and busy. So, lockdown is absolutely perfect for increasing my water intake and training my body to get used to it. I purchased one of those bottles with times and levels printed on the side since I am very visual and need to see goals and progress in order to be successful.

Going downstairs to make coffee is usually the first thing I do when I wake up (I adore good coffee!), but lately, I've been adding drinking the first hour's worth of water to my daily ritual before I have my coffee. The only thing left to do is to be persistent and create the habit. I already have the action (drinking the beverage) and the contextual cue (first thing in the morning before my coffee). How long does it take to develop a habit, though? I hear you say, "21 days," is it true or is that just wishful thinking? According to studies, it can take anywhere from 18 to 254 days to create a habit and alter behaviour, but on average it takes 66 days (Lally, Van Jaarsveld, Potts and Wardle, 2009).

The phrase "21 days" actually relates to plastic surgery and changing one's appearance and is taken from a book written by Dr. Maxwell Maltz in 1960. He didn't state it as a proposition; rather, he only describes the figure as an observable metric. These, along with numerous other often noticed phenomena, according to the author, "tend to suggest that it takes at least roughly 21 days for an old mental image to dissipate and a new one to gel." Despite the fact that more than 30 million copies of the book have been sold and 21 days is commonly believed to be true, it is a hoax!

The length of time it takes for habits to emerge might vary depending on a number of circumstances, which is why the range is so wide. How long it takes for people to create a habit truly relies on how difficult the activity is and how quickly they adjust.

Simple actions with readily available routine cues, like taking a glass of water before breakfast, can easily develop into habits. However, if the aim is to perform 50 sit-ups when you get out of bed or go for a run before breakfast, these actions are likely to take longer to become ingrained since there are more variables that can influence behaviour change. The main element is motivation! Going downstairs to get a glass of water is simple, and even if you don't feel like drinking it, you can still manage to do so without too much difficulty. As a result, it rapidly becomes a habit. However, going for a run or exercising involves far more work and will demand much more deliberate thought and motivation until you do it automatically!

So that you may boost your motivation and succeed in forming habits that will yield results, we need to create a mindset that will give you the call to action. We're going to look at some mindset hacks to do this.

Hack #1: Be certain of your objectives!

You should have created a statement outlining what you REALLY want to accomplish by this point since we discussed goal-setting in Chapter 1 of this book. You ought to have thought about what is significant to you, what you plan to improve, and as a result, what you CAN and WANT to accomplish. If you haven't already, go back and read Chapter 1 and then continue.

Write that statement here…

If your objective is to lose weight or body fat, it's likely that you're actually trying to recreate a happier time in your past. Since it's much simpler to visualise your results when they are you, this is a tremendously effective tool for motivation. I recently looked over some old progress photos I had taken on one of my old phones. It turns out that I was in very good form in 2012, so I'm using that as my current benchmark. Now that I have that image saved to my phone, I can use it as a benchmark to compare my current measurements and photos to my ideal image each month.

Make sure you've chosen a realistic role model for someone you want to resemble if your goal is to increase muscle or size.

In either case, be certain of what it is that you want to accomplish. It is possible to attain goals with a concentrated and clear vision; however, if there are too many unknowns or you frequently change your mind, your chances of success are significantly reduced. If the change is significant and abrupt, divide it into manageable stages so that each stage has a specific goal that must be met before going on to the next. Rome wasn't built in a day, so if you're serious about making a change that will last a lifetime, stick with the process and have patience; the end result will be worthwhile.

Keep the target in close proximity to you, whether it's a photo of how you want to appear, a picture of a piece of clothes you want to look fantastic in, a set of measurements you want to attain, or a bodyfat percentage figure. You should review your objective each day, check in with yourself, and think about why you want to achieve it and what it means to you. You can go to it whenever you need a good nudge in the right direction or a good reminder of why you're making the decisions you are.

Hack# 2: Make a good connection with your objective!

You are aware of your objective, the reasons for setting it, your motivation for working toward it, and the significance of success for you. I want you to picture how it will feel when you succeed now. The way you'll feel on the inside How will you feel when you finally achieve your ideal appearance? How will it feel to wake up every day knowing that you are in the physique you have desired since setting your goal? Hold onto that sensation! We're going to apply it each time we have to make a challenging decision. I want you to pause, take a deep breath, and consider your objective and how you'll feel once you've reached it each time you feel tested, whether it's losing motivation to exercise or abandoning your food plan. Then, I want you to consider whether your decision will be worthwhile.

Clearly, if you've been working out hard and your body is signalling that you need a break, you should pay attention to it. The hack is mainly intended to prevent you from going off the waggon and abandoning your training/eating plan, so skipping the occasional training session or occasionally overindulging in food is not the end of the world.

Achieving your objective will ultimately be determined by whether you truly desire it. If it truly matters to you, this notion will motivate you to work out or refrain from eating the cake.

We're working toward a goal here; we're taking charge of our bodies and how we approach food and drink so that we may feel comfortable in our own flesh. When you do indulge in something from your lifestyle that you have been limiting, it will also improve the experience.

We are aware that when we can have something without doing any work, the enjoyment wears off over time and it becomes less thrilling or delightful. The same holds true with food, particularly sugar, wherein a greater intake blunts our response to the brain's release of reward hormones, requiring us to consume more to feel the same level of satisfaction. We will appreciate the experience of having it and make the most of the hormone release and the favourable effects it has on mood and pleasure if we are more selective about when we allow ourselves to have it. In reference to my passion of going out for coffee, I have the ideal example of this. I found myself getting cake every time I went to a coffee shop after visiting New Zealand and being introduced to real coffee and cake (thanks Warren). Other than the fact that I loved it, or at least thought I did, there is no justification for it. By consuming it frequently, I also began to consume an increasing amount of sweet foods, which decreased my hormone response and enjoyment.

If you think back on your personal experiences, I'm sure you'll agree that there is a distinct difference between mass-produced cake seen at chain coffee shops and cake made by independent bakeries. It definitely wasn't or isn't worth it if you combine that with the guilt you felt for eating it while "trying to eat better." Here's where our mindset and mental processes come into play; I'm not going to tell you that every time you want cake, you should think about your objective and how you feel and say no, but rather that you should ask yourself whether what you're going to experience is worthwhile. Therefore, if I go to a local coffee shop and the cake is "homemade" and it looks amazing, I know I will appreciate the flavour and make the most of the experience, so I'll have a piece and not feel guilty at all since I'm confident in my choice and think it's worthwhile. To keep on track, I may always experiment with my calorie intake and cut back elsewhere in the day.

When I go to a chain restaurant with friends, though, and am given a cake, I am pleased to decline because I know it won't taste as wonderful as it looks and is therefore not worth it. I prefer to refer to this as "owning your choices," when you are certain that you are making the best decisions because you have taken into account all the relevant information. Since you don't have to feel guilty because you are in control, this style of thinking is essential for advancement.

We've gotten off topic a bit, but you're getting effectively two hacks for the price of one there! When faced with a decision, you will connect with your objective, experience it, consider the circumstances, and then determine whether it is worthwhile to you or not.

Hack# 3: Become a social advocate for your objective!

This will show whether you're sincere about your objective and ready to share it with others. You can't undervalue the influence of social commitment since it intensifies the strain, the suspense, and the dread of failing. Now, depending on your mentality and the type of person you are, this might either inspire you or terrify you. We've covered that topic very thoroughly up to this point, so you should know who you are and if you'll survive on this or perish. You decide how public you want to make it, of course, but you must at least discuss your aspirations with someone close to you, even if it's only the folks you live with. You should make your public announcement in front of your fridge, but don't just stand inside and tell everyone who opens the door to do so! Create a progress report for yourself and post it on the refrigerator. Include your milestone goals leading up to the major goal as well as a monthly date for taking your measurements.

Put whatever you intend to track where it will be visible to you every day and to people in your immediate support network. This is a terrific approach to push yourself if you need accountability since even if no one comments on it, you know they will have seen it and will notice if you're making improvement or not. More importantly, you will notice it, so whenever you don't feel like getting out of bed, all you have to do is glance over to see how far you've come and how close you are to reaching your objective.

Hack# 4: Own your decisions!

When faced with a novel option or circumstance, we automatically experience emotion. It's most likely to be either awe, fear, or exhilaration. When presented with a challenge, we either think of all the reasons why we can't do it or aren't bothered to do it right now or we immediately say yes out of enthusiasm before even considering what or how we're going to accomplish something. After our initial instinctual response, the rational part of our brain takes over and considers the circumstances, the facts, and our past experiences to actually decide what to do or how to do it.

The same is true when it comes to eating; we either get thrilled and say yes without thinking about the consequences, or we say no because we don't feel like it (even if we should really have it).

In light of all of this, we now understand that we should let our intuitive emotions some time to pass before letting logic and rational thought take over before responding when faced with enticing food or deciding when or if to exercise. After you've used some of the hacks you've learned thus far, perhaps.

No matter what happens, YOU MUST OWN YOUR CHOICE! You must feel at ease with your decisions if you don't want to go down the path of bitterness if you say no or guilt if you eat that slice of cake.

Having gone through your decision-making process, you've either concluded that your goal is too vital or that the experience isn't worth it, so take that into consideration when you say no. The most crucial aspect of this situation is that you've made the decision to refuse. You're not refusing anything because you "can't," but rather because you don't want it. In contrast, if you choose to say yes, you shouldn't feel awful about it because you are in charge of the choice. You have already gone through the decision-making process, so you can be confident that the experience will be worthwhile and that you can make adjustments to make up for it. James Smith, a controversial fitness expert, uses an excellent analogy when he compares calorie counting to having a daily budget. You alter your remaining budget to get through the rest of the day when you "buy" something (eat or drink). To this, I would add that at the end of the day, you are either on budget (achieving your goal), under budget (having extra calories), or over budget (owing money). As a result, you can base your budget for the following day on these three outcomes and what you need to accomplish after today.

You don't have to sacrifice anything and you can have whatever you want; you just need to decide if it's worth it and how you'll adjust things to make up for it. This is the key to owning your choices and maintaining the proper mindset. For instance, if your daily goal is to walk 10k steps but you only manage 5k, you can always strive for 15k steps the following day or an additional 1k over the course of five days. You may prevent feeling guilty by taking responsibility for your decisions and having a detailed strategy on how to apply them to your week and stay on track. You won't feel defeated, and you won't abandon everything and start over from scratch. It can mean the difference between making progress steadily and giving up once more because it is a much better state of mind to be in.

Hack# 5: Enjoy your victories!

Be careful to recognise and appreciate each of your accomplishments, whether it's reaching a goal or finishing a tough workout.

They all count! Just keep in mind that every step you take brings you closer to your objective and represents improvement over where you were before, so give yourself a pat on the back.

It's also crucial that you take advantage of the chance to acknowledge your wise decisions, particularly if you were put to the test while doing so. Positive reinforcement can help motivate people and improve their learned behaviours. You've probably witnessed this all your life, from your parents praising you for learning something new to your school recognising your work with a good grade to your employer rewarding you with promotions or incentives. Rewarding work or admirable behaviour helps us feel good and motivates us to repeat it in order to achieve more in the future. It's up to you how much self-rewarding you want to do. I would advise that giving yourself some internal encouragement and a metaphorical pat on the back is sufficient, but if you want to treat yourself to a fiver or an extra 15 minutes in bed the following morning every time you make a good decision, go for it! Whatever it is, make sure you stop to think, acknowledge your accomplishment, and give yourself some credit. This will help you adopt positive behaviour, which will make those decisions simpler.

Consider your celebration strategy and, in particular, the objectives you will hit. It's probably not a good idea to celebrate reaching your weekly weight reduction goal by going on a weekend binge and eating everything you want if it's tracking day and you weigh yourself and find that you've succeeded. However, it might be a good idea to treat yourself to something you want or will enjoy. It would be even better if the reward had nothing to do with food or drink. Instead of using success as an excuse to unwind and take your foot off the gas, we must harness its positive aspects and use them to improve our motivation.

Rewards should increase in magnitude as milestones and successes do. When you reach your overall goal for weight/fat loss, for instance, you could treat yourself to a shopping spree. After all, you might need new clothes if you're smaller than you were previously. However, you can decide to treat yourself to something more expensive than you normally would, perhaps a brand or look you've been eyeing. Giving yourself the carrot of a reward in addition to reaching the aim itself just increases the drive to continue being consistent and moving forward. Then, for maximum motivation, we'll discuss internal and extrinsic rewards. Consider your desires and include them into your plan.

Chapter Six
Make your Plan

As I hinted to before, our motivation may be impacted by the fact that we tend to think and act emotionally first before using our reasoning and logical brain regions. When we give our brain a new goal that will require work and apparent sacrifice, it immediately responds with negative ideas! It requires a clear understanding of how you intend to accomplish this goal, including the steps necessary, how you intend to carry them out, and how long it will take.

The time is not right for unknowns! So far, we have learned more about you and figured out the who, what, and how oftens (I don't know if that's a word, but it is now!) Therefore, we theoretically have a plan; we just need to flesh it out. If you're listening to the book, get your paper again because we're going to make your strategy now.

What exercise are you going to do?

What days are you going to do it?

Are you going to do it by yourself? With a friend? In a class? With a trainer?

Are you doing it for fun or are you going to track your workouts/sessions?

With that in place, you can be sure that you now understand what you need to do physically to achieve your objectives. Let's apply this concept to your eating now.

How many calories do you need each day?

This number can be obtained by utilising a macronutrient calculator. There are some extremely helpful websites that ask for your data (height, weight, age), followed by your level of activity, and then provide you with the daily caloric and macronutrient requirements (carbs, protein, and fat).

Calories –

To reduce weight or fat, you must have a calorie deficit; therefore, as you lose weight, you will need less calories to maintain your progress. Keep this in mind whenever you lose weight. On the other hand, when your weight rises, you'll require more calories if you're trying to put on muscle.

Protein –

The macronutrient you want to focus on the most is protein. It not only aids in the recovery and expansion of your exercise-damaged muscles, but it also helps you feel satisfied for a longer period of time. Therefore, it performs a crucial role in assisting you in becoming slimmer even if you are not weight exercising.

Carbs –

In attempts to lose weight or fat, carbs are always the bad guy. There is no question that reducing or eliminating carbohydrates from your diet can lead you to lose weight and fat, but this is only true if you also make significant calorie reductions, which will result in a calorie deficit. But realistically, it's impossible to be content while adhering to a low-carb diet. Why would you give up some of the best-tasting meals in existence, which are carbohydrate-rich? We require carbohydrates to function during exercise and in daily life because they are the body's main source of energy. They can be reduced to sugar in their most basic form, so be mindful of how much sugar is in the meals you consume. We discussed how eating a lot of sugar will have a blunting effect on the release of the reward hormone. Therefore, if you often consume too many sugary carbs, you'll crave them even more to achieve the reward, which will probably result in eating too many calories!

Fat –

Don't be afraid of fat; ingesting too many calories causes weight gain rather than eating fat. The body uses it and uses it in cellular activity. So, go ahead and indulge in whatever you want in its full fat form as long as you stay under your calorie budget and your target weight (but avoid fizzy drinks!).

Are you going to bulk cook meals for the week or cook daily?

Do you need to plan whole days, or can you do it per meal on the day?

Do you need to take your own food, or can you trust yourself to buy food out?

Will you have similar meals each week or do you need lots of variety?

Can you create your own eating plan, or do you need help from a professional?

Can you cook or do you need to take lessons?

A sincere question: Do you know how to prepare the meals you need or want, or are you used to throwing manufactured food into the oven? If you fall into the latter category, learning to cook could completely shift your trajectory.

Therefore, we now have a framework for how you will achieve your fitness and dietary goals. MyFitnessPal is a great app for tracking your food intake because it has a barcode scanner and an extensive food and drink database that makes tracking a breeze. I think theirs is frequently greater, so be sure to set your own calories and modify the macros to your goal.

Every time your weight fluctuates, don't forget to modify your calorie and macro intake. Even though tracking isn't required forever, it is a good idea to do so as you adjust to your daily caloric intake. In order to hold yourself accountable and determine what you did to be successful or what you need to alter if you are not, I would also suggest doing it while you are working towards a goal. If you want to progress, you must have correct data to work with, therefore be fully honest with your tracking as only you will see it.

Chapter Seven
Create Energy for Motivation

Once you've decided that you're going to start, it's very usual to become thrilled (I use the phrase loosely) about getting in shape. You decide how you're going to exercise and start considering how you're going to alter your diet all of a sudden feel motivated to take action.

When you start the day with a healthy breakfast, decline the cake offered to you at work, then go for a run when you get home, day one is complete! On day two, you simply repeat the entire procedure. On day three, it's a little more difficult, but you manage! On day four, you had a decent breakfast, but you forgot to pack a lunch. As a result, you wind up at the store and buy whatever is nearby. After a long day, you go home and realise that you really ought to go for that run, but you're feeling lethargic from lunch and just don't feel like it. You postpone doing it until tomorrow. That's when you stumble; your motivation fails you, and tomorrow also doesn't come. You're back at ground zero after eating, sleeping, and repeating.

How can we prevent this from happening, then? Why are you required to perform both at once? If you're just getting started, you already have a lot of work to do to start eating healthier or exercising more. Why therefore take on two significant issues at once? Yes, maintaining a healthy diet and increasing your exercise will help you achieve your goals, but it doesn't mean you have to start doing them both at once.

How do you feel when you begin a new endeavour and start to succeed? You must feel good about it. You appreciate the sensation of accomplishment and are inspired to do more!

With this in mind, you should be picky about where you start when you have a list of activities you need to do or goals you want to achieve. Choose the endeavour that will bring you great success quickly. These minor victories will lift your spirits, make you feel like you're progressing well, and increase your confidence in your ability to succeed. You feel more inspired and prepared to accomplish more as a result of this.

You can channel that vigour and use it to launch the subsequent stage. Returning to the exercise example, let's put this in perspective. Determine which of your tasks offers you the most satisfaction first. Which would you choose: changing your food habits or increasing your exercise?

Always take the option that will lead to success for you the quickest. Utilize this drive to gain momentum before beginning the other component. You'll then be prepared to smash your goals on all fronts and look for those outcomes with your motivation on fire!

You set yourself up for the best possibility of success by being deliberate and clever about how you launch your new way of life. You'll not only advance physically more quickly, but you'll also keep your motivation strong and prevent yourself from slacking off. Though it is a relatively straightforward concept, it has great potential.

Chapter Eight
Make Plan to Fail

Now that we know how you expect to accomplish your objectives, we need to establish a failure plan. This sounds quite strange, don't you think? But it is true! If you don't prepare for failure, missing a goal or seeing less progress than anticipated may come as a shock to you and may cause you to veer off course. I want you to have a plan instead so that if something goes wrong and you miss a goal, you'll know how to handle it rather than allowing it to throw your thinking and your attention off course! Failure is an opportunity for growth; if you have a plan and have been keeping track of your activities, you have all the information you need to draw lessons from the setback and figure out how to prevent it from happening again.

Let's use a weigh-in as an example; you set a goal to lose 1 lb, but when you get on the scale, you discover that you have gained 1 lb. This would be sufficient to send Sandra from Fat Fighters into a downward spiral of self-loathing and failure-blaming. Or else, she'll complain about the lousy software for disappointing her. She'll then have two options: she'll punish herself by cutting calories, starving herself, and feeling terrible, or she'll choose the other route, give up, and eat anything she's been yearning! But since you've been wise and have made plans for setbacks, you don't need to do that. Armed with your data, you can assess your past behaviour to determine if you consumed too many calories or weren't active enough. The method can then be repeated at your following tracking point once you have revised your plan for the coming week and adjusted the variables.

With this method, you are always in charge and can deal with any obstacles with ease since you have thought through how you would handle them. This is crucial for your motivation and sense of self-worth, and you should apply these ideas to all of your endeavours. Punishing yourself must be avoided at all costs! According to B.F. Skinner's research, negative reinforcement has similar effects to positive reinforcement in terms of its ability to alter behaviour. A child is more likely to be afraid to approach dogs in the future out of fear of repetition if their first encounter with a dog results in the dog being aggressive or even biting them. Therefore, all incentive to be with dogs is gone.

If, despite your best efforts during the week, you gained weight and punish yourself for it based solely on your feelings, it's likely that your motivation will decline out of fear of failing once more. Therefore, we eliminate "feeling" from the equation and only use the information at hand! No punishment is required; just a few modest changes and a strategy for the coming week!

We currently live in a society where those who have "influence" over us—not just Instagram celebrities, but also esteemed friends and family—project flawless lives and abundant success on social media. We seldom ever see any of the struggle that went into getting there; instead, we always seem to see the glory. When trying to lose weight or reduce body fat, a progression graph almost never has a straight line as the goal. For instance, in the image below, I've included a screenshot of my Boditrax log from the gym, which shows muscle mass.

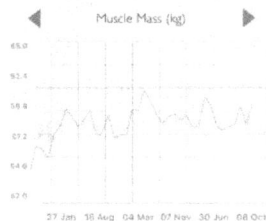

As you can see, there are a lot of gains and losses, all of which contribute to improvement when compared to the beginning, but there is also a lot of variation depending on how precise and reliable my tracking, eating, and exercising were.

Congratulations on achieving your goal of losing 1 lb per week for 12 weeks; it's a remarkable accomplishment! However, if you don't, don't worry about it; it doesn't say anything negative about you, your skills, or your work. Life can and certainly will get in the way at some point, but why should you lose out on a birthday, a holiday, or an unexpectedly warm weekend that shouts for a BBQ? If you're on a transformation plan, I'd advise you to schedule events like the ones I've listed in your time frame map. This will enable you to take them into account and alter your calories and exercise levels to account for them in advance. If, however, they arise at the last minute, you may still make accommodations.

The most crucial thing of all is that you have the mindset to maintain control and understand that even though it's a momentary setback, it doesn't preclude you from achieving your objective. You have techniques to help you get back on track.

Smaller goals that lead to the major goal are great because they not only keep us motivated and hold us accountable, but they also offer us a real-time image of where we are so we can plan ahead to see if we're on schedule.

We have the luxury of getting another week if we need it because we aren't Instagram celebrities or magazine cover models.

Give yourself plenty of time if your physical goal is a vacation! I had had a client ask me if I could help them achieve results two WEEKS before their vacation when I used to work on the gym floor.

However, this is merely a backup plan; in reality, throughout a metamorphosis, you want these situations to be as seldom as possible. You might get away with one every 4-6 weeks, but if you have blowouts every week, I'm afraid you'll need to add on a lot of time to reach your goal. It all boils down to knowing yourself, your lifestyle, and what you're willing to change, as well as being realistic about your goal. You realise you'll need to be pretty tight with yourself the other 6 days to make room for it and still achieve your goals if you want to go out and drink once a week every week. The topics we reviewed in this chapter apply to you if you go out, say, once a month.

In the end, this is your book, your goals, and your life. I'm empowering you with the knowledge you need to create a strategy that will work for you. Simply being realistic and honest with yourself will do.

Anyway, enough about failure; it's a gloomy term with gloomy implications, so I want to present you with a different perspective.

Chapter Nine
Tracking and Self-image

I have a lot of feelings regarding both tracking and self-image, and they are both HUGE concerns for me. They have the potential to significantly affect your mood and sense of self, and they can also cause you to get fixated on the outcomes. I've dealt with it with my clients and lived with it, so hopefully I can help you with it today.

Let's start by discussing weight. Who is actually interested in your weight? Do you carry a set of scales that show your weight to everyone wherever you go? If you succeed in reaching your target, will your best buddy greet you with "oh my god, you look —kg" or "wow, you look great"? Everyone says, "Oh, I want to lose weight," but do you really? The world is so obsessed with body weight. Put down your keyboards, warriors; if I were to be correct, you could lose 10 pounds without actually changing anything about how you looked (obviously, you'd notice, but this is just an assumption). or if you could maintain your weight while losing a waist size, which option would you pick? Shape alteration is really what you're after! You don't have to be narcissistic to appreciate it when others notice your accomplishments and compliment you on them; it's a great lift, and if you put in the effort, you deserve it!

Because of this, I advise against choosing a specific figure as your "target weight" since it has no real significance. However, you do need to be aware of your weight because we utilise it to calculate your calorie needs. I also advise you to weigh yourself each week, but you should just do so to see if you've made progress, not necessarily to determine how much. Positive progress is always welcome, but it also serves as confirmation that your course of action is the right one. Keep in mind that we are utilising this for accountability and that it also influences our data; we are not fixated on the number because it is unimportant to us. It's important to weigh yourself consistently, therefore attempt to weigh yourself at the same time every day in the same location and on a hard surface.

I prefer to weigh myself after drinking my first bottle of water since I use bioelectrical impedance scales and want to ensure that my hydration is at its peak for a more accurate measurement. To obtain a more accurate picture of my progress, I therefore ensure that I am consistent each week. This isn't the gold standard of measuring and it's not the most exact, but it's accessible and gives me a good notion, and it's for my own personal objective, so a rough estimate is OK! I'm mainly interested in the body fat percentage in my readings because that is what my transformation objective is predicated on. I don't care about my weight, but I would like to get leaner because it will improve how I look.

I monitor both of them every week since they provide the information I need to modify my eating habits during the week. I know I'm eating enough calories if my weight has fallen, but if my body fat % hasn't, I know I need to eat more protein throughout the course of the next week to maintain and grow my muscle so I can get leaner.

So those are the measurements I gather and track each week. As part of my progress tracking, I will also take measurements of my chest, arms, waist, lower belly, and legs each month. I lift weights with the goal of becoming leaner, so I want to make sure that my chest and arms remain the same size or even increase, while also losing belly fat and maintaining a small waist size. I only do this once a month since we don't typically notice changes in measures as rapidly as we do with weight changes. My body fat % should give me a good notion of how I'm doing with muscle, but the measurements provide me information I can use in my workouts. It might decide how I divide up my workouts, if I work out a certain body region more frequently, etc.

I don't get too wrapped up in the figures; they're just more evidence that supports or informs my plan. I'll then take two shots of the progress each month, one from the front and one from the side. Again, consistency is key here. Take photos in the same location with as much consistency in the lighting as you can. I compare using the images since until you can actually see the difference, numbers don't mean too lot. But bodily dysmorphia and low self-esteem are right here, with potential for enormous issues.

Body dysmorphia, which is categorised as a mental health issue, is characterised by excessive self-consciousness. By that definition, you'd assume that nearly everyone in the world possesses it! It goes beyond that, frequently causing you to obsess over a particular body component you believe needs improvement and even to perceive your body differently than other people do.

Bodybuilders frequently run the danger of exhibiting body dysmorphic characteristics, especially if they compete. Even if no one else has seen it, as their body changes and gets better, they will move on to the next area that they believe to be small or fat. Due to the emergence of films and tales addressing the problem, it has also recently been referred to as "Bigorexia." The illness is fueled by a skewed perception of one's own body, which can result in eating disorders and other mental health issues, such as depression.

These characteristics can also be found in those who have begun and partially completed a weight/fat loss change. They will also examine themselves and identify other areas they believe want development. These persons are most at risk of developing eating disorders as a result of continuing to restrict their caloric intake in an effort to lose weight.

Not everyone who exhibits symptoms will go on to develop eating disorders and depression because there are different levels of every ailment, and it is manageable. This is one of the reasons I document my progress using a mix of weekly weigh-ins, monthly measurements, and monthly progress photos. I can support that with the measurements and scales' data if I don't notice a significant change in the images. This aids in mental satisfaction and prevents me from worrying excessively about my appearance or making plans to exercise more or eat less.

So, here is the closest thing to a sob tale from me that you'll ever get, just in case you hadn't figured out that I have body dysmorphia. I'm not telling you this to win your sympathy; instead, I'm telling you this to give you a real-world example of how it works. Since I manage my illness using the data, it doesn't really affect me on a daily basis anymore.

I believe I made the commitment to get a six-pack for the summer for a period of more than ten years. To be fair to myself, one summer when I was about 16 or 17, I believe I came very close before I self-sabotaged and feared that I was losing too much muscle and becoming too thin. This turned out to be a recurring pattern or battle for me over a long period of time, and it still is to some level. I've fluctuated between wanting to grow muscle, adding some bodyfat, and being anxious about gaining weight once more, to decreasing weight to get rid of the bodyfat I'd accumulated, feeling like I was also losing my muscle mass, and then repeating the cycle. This is demonstrated in real time by the muscle mass progress graph I used earlier in this book.

It varies considerably from day to day as well; on some days, you may feel as like you are making progress, but on other days, you may think, "Oh god, that looks dreadful, I need to do x, y, and z." This is why having a detailed plan that you comprehend and are confident in is crucial. You can take a deep breath, allow your rational brain take over, and remind yourself that you're working toward a plan that will help you achieve the outcomes you're after when you look in the mirror and your emotional brain starts to worry.

My bodyfat percentage is still far higher than I would like it to be as of this writing. I recently found some old phones while organising some things, and after reading through them, I was able to determine when I last felt pretty healthy, which was in 2012! Since then, gaining weight, including muscle and fat, losing it, then gaining it back, and so forth, has been a perpetual cycle. The only problem is that every time I lost it, I didn't drop as much as I had gained initially, and over the past eight years, my bodyfat percentage has slowly risen. I believe I was aware of it, but since I've put on a fair bit of muscle, I was sort of okay with it. In fact, I believe that body dysmorphia can also have an adverse effect. (This is entirely my own rhetoric; I haven't looked into it in any way; I'm just writing what's on my mind.) Yeah, ok, pretty good chest, arms, and shoulders; might need some work on the tummy, but not too awful, I thought as I stared in the mirror. The general rule of thumb is that you're doing okay if your chest protrudes more than your tummy. The truth, however, is that by allowing me to remain in my comfort zone, I was able to increase the amount of fat on my lower abs and around my obliques (commonly referred to as "love handles"), which has only made me unhappy.

Now that I think about it, I see that I advocate for being at ease with who you are, and I just stated that I was at a point where I felt good about myself, so there shouldn't be a problem. But you also need to be honest with yourself about your behaviours and how they affect your body. I am better than most at knowing what I should do and how my actions will affect my body. I know that if I choose foods that are high in sugar and simple carbohydrates, which I find to be very easy to do, I will gain weight. I need to eat enough protein to preserve the bulk I now have because I am aware of how much my level of muscle mass can vary. Because I had persuaded myself that I was fine exactly the way I was, I was very slack with my eating and drinking during the time I just stated. As a result, I gained weight until it was pointed out to me.

I am a rugby referee, and I have had the good fortune to officiate matches here in the UK and all around the world. When you reach a respectable level, there is a lot of pressure to appear "beautiful," so when I started to acquire weight around my belly and hips, it was quickly brought up to me. This may seem strange to you. We meet once a month as a training officer for a local referee society. People at these meetings will often comment on my weight gain or loss, and I don't think they realise how much of an effect that has on me. But I have to admit that I have come to understand over the past few months that they are entirely correct. To be fully honest with you, the way my t-shirts fit on me made it clear that I had a hand's worth of fat on my hips and lower tummy. Yes, my chest and shoulders could handle some weight gain, but the lower tummy and hips were beginning to interfere with how the t-shirts hung.

I decided to change it after giving myself a reality check. Although this may seem like another cycle, I actually have a completely different perspective and outlook on what I'm trying to accomplish this time around. In fact, this thinking and outlook served as the inspiration for this book.

I've been examining how to manage your diet and exercise in a way that promotes a healthy mental relationship. By that, I mean strategies for managing your eating habits while avoiding obsession and emotional ups and downs as you lose and gain weight. It's impossible to maintain consistency all the time because there are constant, natural changes in lifestyle based on a variety of factors, such as events in your life or situations that may cause you to lose focus or alter your priorities. We must acknowledge that there will be periods when we are more focused and other times when we are more relaxed.

Thus, it is extremely strong and crucial to prepare our minds for this by realising that we are in control and that we can simply change things when we realise that we need to!

Instead of fluctuating between boom and bust, we just rise and fall above and below a constant maintenance line. When we reach the levels we desire, we can let our tracking slip, and if we fall short of our goals, we can take it back up and move on. This doesn't entail making radical adjustments or "beginning another diet," just being more aware of what we're eating once more and realigning with how much is required to maintain the level we desire. This is now a way of life; it gives you the flexibility to lead a comfortable life in control! Understanding your body's needs, what you can get away with, and how to make changes to get your desired outcome are all important. You can always get back on track by applying the tips and principles we've covered in this book whenever you stray from where you'd like to be.

We also need to learn to appreciate the process so that we may continue to eat the foods we love even when we are on a calorie-restricted diet! The main distinction is that you will tweak it to accommodate a certain meal or beverage. I think that learning to like food also helps you have a better relationship with it. I discover that it also aids in my decision-making regarding whether or not I will actually have it. If it doesn't live up to my expectations, I'll know it's not worth the calories the next time and won't bother, but if I do appreciate it, I'll look forward to it and make the most of it the next time I have it.

A fruit scone with clotted cream and jam is my personal favourite. I bought some fresh, delicious scones from the grocery store, so I added some clotted cream and jam to my daily calorie allowance. The taste was incredible, so full of flavour and just as excellent as I had hoped, plus it really complimented the coffee, so it checked all of my boxes. I made a coffee and went to sit in the garden. I adore the sensation of enjoying delicious food and a good cup of coffee while sitting in the sun in my garden, so whenever I get that experience, I make sure to fully immerse myself in it. I also eat slowly to maximise the flavours and savour every bite. It completely justifies the calories!

Even better, I know how to plan my meals and drinks such that I can still enjoy these things even if I'm watching my calorie intake. This is the discovery I want to share with you: limitation doesn't have to be difficult or mean giving up everything you enjoy; it just has to be taken into account. To keep within your limits, you simply need to be aware of what and how much you're eating so that you can determine what else you're having during the day.

Look how easily I became sidetracked when discussing food! Having said that, it can improve your happiness and general welfare to know that you don't have to live a limited life and can still do what you want without feeling guilty. A strong and upbeat mid-set is essential for wellbeing as well as success. Take a moment to stand back, take a deep breath, consider the amount of progress you've made, and decide to be happy about it since it's far too simple to become obsessed with results and how we appear.

I want you to start with the positives whenever you take images or measurements before you do anything else! Choose an area in which you've made headway, acknowledge the difference, and feel good about it. Then, because you're approaching it with a positive mindset based on the success you've already made, an area you still want to improve in won't seem that horrible. As a result, it simply becomes the next area of concentration.

I want you to keep these ideas in mind because they are all very helpful for developing a strong attitude that emphasises achievement and growth so that you may keep getting better. We believe in encouraging and supporting ourselves, not humiliating and punishing ourselves because that doesn't fit with our way of thinking. We are a strong, positive, and forward-thinking group of individuals, and we WILL achieve our goals!

Chapter Ten
Bringing it about

Well done if you've made it this far; you should now be much better equipped to obtain the outcomes you actually desire. This chapter serves as a recap and a final dose of motivation before sending you out into the world to make it happen!

I hope you've had many opportunity to pause and consider who you are as a person as you've read the book to identify your needs, preferences, and get a sense of what works best for you. I'll repeat it again: in order for you to advance throughout your life, this knowledge is very essential.

You should already have a lot of ideas about how you want to exercise, when you want to exercise, and who you want to exercise with (if anyone). Additionally, you should have plans for changing your diet. Keep in mind that you don't have to stop eating your favourite foods; instead, you just need to alter how much or perhaps how frequently you consume them.

Additionally, you ought to be very clear about what your objective is. Do you still want to lose weight, or is your real objective to change your body's composition? Do you truly care what the scale says, or would you rather feel and look good? Always be detailed when setting goals so that you can add steps to your plan and have a clear understanding of what you hope to accomplish.

We are aware that in order to feel fulfilled and think logically, our brain need clarity and understanding of the plan. (Although I have simplified that remark, it still puts things into perspective for the average person to understand.) By doing this, you'll be able to make decisions more quickly and easily when you're faced with tough options. One of the most important lessons I want you to learn from this book is to own your choices, which is why I didn't say "better choices." We must eliminate shame from your workout and diet decisions if we want to be effective and safeguard your mental health! Your viewpoint will change, and you'll stay on the path to success, if you know what you're doing and are confident in your decisions. having faith in your ability to simply modify your plan moving forward to protect yourself and stay on track, even if you overindulge or miss a workout!

The other important point I want you to remember is to treat your daily calorie budget like a budget. This is yet another important element in changing your perspective and your relationship with food. Additionally, it makes the process much simpler to comprehend! Knowing that you can control your caloric intake changes the way you approach food, especially when trying to lose weight. Although cutting calories is a need if you want to lose weight, working within a budget seems much more motivating than following a calorie-restricted diet. Additionally, it's much simpler to comprehend when balancing out a week's worth of consumption, especially if you've had a day of overindulgence. In order to get yourself "back into the black" after going all out and indulging in takeout, a few beers, and other indulgences, you just tweak your budget for the following day or a few days to make up for the excess calories you consumed on that particular day. By doing this, you may remain adaptable in life and yet achieve your goals and advance. This is the key to maintaining control, avoiding guilt, and preventing emotional chaos.

Plus, we've also equipped you with 5 motivation hacks to help you make choices and continue to progress. They are...

Hack #1: Be certain of your objectives!

Hack #2: Make a good connection with your objective!

Hack #3: Become a social advocate for your objective!

Hack #4: Own your decisions!

Hack # 5: Enjoy your victories!

Therefore, by this point, you ought to have posed a lot of questions to yourself and assembled a list of responses. We've given you a target, we've looked at how you're going to get there, and we've added 5 hacks to your toolbox to help you get motivated, pick up speed, and keep moving forward. Now all you have to do is put your plan into action.

The time to reach out, learn what you need to learn, and fill those gaps is NOW if you require expert assistance. But be sure to get going RIGHT NOW, TODAY! Don't be one of those persons who creates a plan then waits for the "perfect time" to implement it. RIGHT NOW is the time! Make a start today by doing AT LEAST one item, such as hiring a trainer, selecting a new lunch, or simply taking an extra stroll. Set those things in motion by releasing your brand-new, optimistic, forward-thinking mindset. As long as you start and keep moving forward, it doesn't matter how slowly you progress.

Make careful to surround oneself with uplifting people as well. Go through your social media feeds and unfollow any accounts that make you feel horrible or post unrealistic images or content, for example. Find people who inspire you and who post information that is valuable to you and moves you to action. You are in control of how you feel in your social spaces and how they help you learn and develop as a person, so go ahead and update your feed to reflect your new outlook.

You may achieve the mental space you require to ignite your motivation and make progress by following all of the instructions throughout the book. You are at an exciting period of your life right now, so take advantage of it and fulfil your long-held goals!

I appreciate you reading my book, and please get in touch with me via my social media accounts to let me know how you're doing and how your new outlook has changed your life!

Best wishes

James Wallace

REFERENCES

Scientific Papers

Atkinson, J.W. (1974) 'the mainstream of achievement-oriented activity' in Atkinson, J.W. And Raynor, J.O. (eds) motivation and achievement, New York, Halstead.

Mcclelland, D. (1961) The achieving society, New York, Free Press.

Mullins, L.J. (2002) managing people in organisations, Milton Keynes, The Open University.

Weiner, B. (1985) 'an attribution theory of achievement motivation and emotion', psychological review, vol.92, pp. 548-73.

Neal DT, Wood W, Labrecque JS, Lally P. How do habits guide behavior? Perceived and actual triggers of habits in daily life. j exp soc psychol. 2012;48:492–498. [google scholar]

Lally P, Wardle J, Gardner B, Psychol health med. 2011 aug; 16(4):484-9. [pubmed]

Phillippa Lally*, Cornelia H. M. Van Jaarsveld, Henry W. W. Potts and Jane Wardle, How are habits formed: modelling habit formation in the real world. European journal of social psychology eur. J. Soc. Psychol. 40, 998–1009 (2010)

www.ingramcontent.com/pod-product-compliance
Lightning Source LLC
Chambersburg PA
CBHW071116030426
42336CB00013BA/2107